Gavin Jamie is a medical doctor who has worked in the National Health Service for over twenty years, for the last eighteen years of that time as a General Practitioner. He has an interest in healthcare informatics and has written extensively in the medical press about the Quality and Outcomes Framework and other subjects related to the accurate entry of medical data.

He also runs a medical data website and is in general practice in Swindon, Wiltshire.

Starting Snomed

A Beginner's Guide to the Snomed CT Healthcare Terminology

Gavin Jamie

To my family,
who wondered what I was doing
and to my former rabbit
who inspired many examples

Contents

Coding Health Data

In 17th century London the civic authorities had a problem that will seem familiar to anybody working in healthcare today. Clerks gathered a lot of information about the population, but there was no easy way to understand it. Every single christening, marriage and death inside the city limits had been recorded by parish clerks since 1538 but no-one actually used the data.

In particular, information on the causes of deaths was not being used effectively, and in an age where much of the population did not have any access to medical services this was pretty much the only information about health that existed. As plague spread through London in final decade of the century it became particularly important to measure death accurately.

To try to make sense of this information, clerks began to publish summarised records of recent deaths in "Bills of Mortality". Each death was placed into a specific category before a total was calculated. These were then published for the authorities, and later the general public to read.

The Bills use a lot of terms that we would not recognise these days. Neither "frighted" or "distracted" would be considered an acceptable cause of death in modern medicine. "Teeth and worms" also seems to have been a surprisingly common cause of death. Even at the time some of these terms were surprising to doctors. It was usual to have the cause of death determined not by a doctor but by "searchers", elderly women who would visit homes after a death to view the body. As in modern times, the quality of the published information was highly dependent on the expertise of the people who collected it in the first place.

Reading the data, John Graunt, a merchant and founder member of the Royal Society, observed that some causes of death affected men more than women. Some varied from season to season whilst others were relatively constant. Although the information is basic, these Bills represented the beginning of the use of statistical methods to examine medical data and using a set of classifications of causes of death. By grouping together similar causes of death, patterns of disease could emerge.

For the next three centuries, death was almost of the only piece of medical data to be recorded in any structured way. Methods of classification and recording improved greatly as the science of statistics developed over that time.

The collection of data for statistical purposes spread around the world alongside other European ideas of government and became a vital part of public health, but the fundamental principle first developed with the Bills of Mortality remained unchanged. In 1893 the International List of Causes of Death was adopted around the world. Now known as the International Classification of Diseases (ICD) it is curated by the World Health Organisation and is used for statistics and research purposes around the globe.

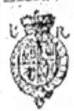

Figure 1: Bill of Mortality from December 1665

The second reason for medical coding was brought about by of the rise of medical insurance in the second half of the twentieth century. Before medical insurance was popularised, a doctor would generally present a bill for payment directly to the patient, or to the next of kin if the doctor had been less successful. But as patients took to medical insurance, insurance companies required itemised bills so that they could compare the price of items between different doctors or hospitals. In the early days of medical insurance, existing methods of coding disease were unhelpful because they looked purely at a diagnosis, rather than the number of operations and treatments the patient had received.

Accurate coding became vital for doctors and hospitals, who wanted to get paid for the work they'd done. Likewise, accurate analysis of these codes was important to insurance companies that wanted to ensure that they were not being overcharged. Often the coding systems for these activities were completely separate from those describing diagnosis. With large sums of money at stake these classifications rapidly developed into sophisticated systems. Examples include OPCS-4 in the UK and ICD-10 Procedure coding (ICD-10-PCS) in the USA.

The last couple of decades of the 20th century brought the rise of the personal computer and its use in patient information collection. Whilst large mainframes had previously assisted with billing or statistical analysis, these new machines could sit on doctors' desks or on the wards. They were primarily used to track patients around the hospital, but their clinical use quickly expanded, and they became extremely effective at communicating the results of laboratory investigations of blood or other samples.

Over time computer systems developed greater capacity to store information about, for example, the medicines that a patient was taking or data such as body temperature or blood pressure, record care plans and to pass messages about patients and their treatment. Much of the time this information was not particularly useful for billing or recording death, but dramatically improved clinicians' capacity to provide care to patients.

An electronic record has several advantages over a conventional paper record. In a well-designed computer system, it is more difficult for the record to become lost. It can be accessed from several different locations at once. An immediate advantage to clinicians using the electronic record is that it can present information in a more helpful and dynamic way: we can easily see all of the information from today – a snapshot of the most up-to-date observations about the patient, as well as their medical history.

The computer could show us how the patient's temperature or blood pressure has changed over time as a table or as a chart. We can automatically generate a summary with only the most significant diagnoses or procedures from the past: say, every operation and all episodes of heart disease but not list every time the patient had a cold or grazed their knee. A specialist could filter the information about heart disease or mental health or anything else appropriate to their speciality.

Like the Bills of Mortality, a modern-day record usually shows just a small part of a patient's medical data in order to produce something that is easily understood. Filtering of information has been done manually for years: for example, summary sheets were maintained in paper records for quick reference. These were often a great relief to a doctor presented with a patient record many inches thick.

To filter a record requires the computer to have some knowledge about the data. If you ask for a chart of the patient's blood pressure over the last week the system needs to know which observations represent a blood pressure measurement and be able to interpret the dates that they were taken.

A more advanced case would be a list of operations which a patient had undergone. The systems need to know which entries in the record are defined as surgery.

Ideally the computer system should also be able to use information about drugs that have been prescribed to show what the patient is currently taking. Just writing out in English sentences is not enough to allow this sort of filtering. We must put this in a form that is understood by the computer.

This could be done by having a separate section of the electronic record for each type of information like columns on a spreadsheet. For very simple records this approach would work well, but it becomes complicated quite quickly. A simple blood count can easily produce 15 types of information; additional tests will push that number up rapidly. Adding extra types of information to the record, such as a new test or procedure, could require a new version of the software which will need to be written, tested and then sent out to users. This is not a small task.

Using a coding system allows information to be recorded in a structured way. Even in a very extensive record, the system can filter data to show only what is relevant. If the same coding system is used by different users, it becomes possible to transfer patient data between systems without any need to re-enter information. There would need to be some extra effort when the information is recorded and coded in the first place, but the advantages should make this worthwhile.

As computer system become more ubiquitous in surgeries and hospitals this communication becomes more important. In my surgery I have programs for patient records, reading letters, ordering blood tests and even printing specimen labels that all have to share patient information.

I also receive information from laboratories and hospital clinics. A common system of recording patient data allows that information to be integrated with the patient record on my computer system, although this is still far from comprehensive.

One of the biggest problems in coding health records are that the advantages of a better system do not always benefit the people who work the hardest to implement and improve systems.

There is a one more way in which systems can help us to use the medical record and pass the advantage to clinicians on the front line: we can teach systems what we mean by a well-coded record. In current systems this is about following relatively simple rules or programs to help a system, for example, give advice about which medications might cause unwanted side effects or interactions. Systems could also advise clinicians about which tests or investigations would be recommended, and alert them to results that might be significant. Guidelines are coded into the computer system to give advice, although the final decision is left to the clinician. This is commonly referred to as decision support.

Such a system could also monitor and even report back on specific treatment plans for individual patients. To do this the computer simply needs to have some idea about the meaning of codes in the clinical record. We would want to be enter a rule such as "Has the patient had an antibiotic?" without having to list every single antibiotic. However, this can only work if the clinical system knows what is, or is not, an antibiotic[1].

Decision support operates using the contents of individual records to give advice in the consulting room, but we can use similar rules to monitor the care of a group of patients – this is the basis of clinical audit. This can be used to monitor patient safety as well as help to ensure that effective treatments are used. For the moment this is not usually what might be called artificial intelligence, although that will surely come in the near future. Whilst well-coded data is not enough to ensure patient safety, it certainly makes it easier for clinicians to monitor the quality of care that is being delivered.

Much of this could be done with the coding systems that we had already. Where diseases had been classified already in order to record causes of death it is pretty easy to go on to use this to record each diagnosis or condition that the patient has. The most common way to do this

---

[1] That is not quite the same as knowing what an antibiotic is

has been the International Classification of Diseases, currently in its eleventh edition (ICD-11).

Similarly, if a patient has a procedure then there are already systems designed to record these for billing purposes. These can be used to record procedures as they have happened and make it possible to have a complete history of procedures that the patient has undergone.

There are limits to that approach, though. We will need additional codes for observations such as lab tests, blood pressure or temperature readings. We might want to record some extra information about how a test is carried out: was the blood pressure measured with a sphygmomanometer (around the arm) or by a sensor in an artery? That can be essential information when interpreting the record. Body temperature can be taken in several different ways and chemistry tests can be performed on various body fluids. All of these will require extra ways of being coded if we want the medical record to be complete.

Snomed CT is a medical terminology system designed to meet the requirements of a modern electronic health record. Its strengths are in recording clinical information in a structured and meaningful way. In the following chapters we will explore how it can be used to do this and produce a medical record that is helpful to clinicians and can contribute to high quality care for patients.

Snomed CT was formed from a merger of previous versions Snomed RT and the UK's Read codes although it has developed significantly since then. For simplicity I will use the word Snomed to refer to Snomed CT.

We will also see how Snomed adds meaning to these codes by allowing them to be defined by their relationships to each other. It is these meanings that can enable automatic systems to intelligently assist the delivery of healthcare.

You don't need to be a computer expert to use Snomed any more than you do to use a cash machine or your mobile phone. This book is aimed at people who are using Snomed to record and retrieve clinical information. Clearly someone has to program the computer in the first place but in a clinical setting we can ignore most of that as being "somebody else's problem". In some systems the coding may not be obvious to most users. The computer will ask for relevant information in a structured way. There will be boxes to fill in and options to select.

The coding system will be more apparent when extracting information from clinical systems or designing templates for data entry. For most of this book we will be looking at how Snomed fits together rather than how the computer deals with this. Things get a little more technical in the later chapters when we talk about moving to Snomed and using it alongside ICD-10 or other coding and reporting systems, but you should be ready for it by then! If you want to go further there are links to further information and courses at the end of the book.

Similarly, I won't assume any great knowledge of medical terminology. Where I do talk about specific conditions these should be familiar to anyone with even the most passing interest in health.

Snomed has been developed as an international project and continues to be owned and run by a non-profit organisation, Snomed International. Individual countries can join the organisation to introduce the use of Snomed into that country: currently there are 30 countries who are members. Organisations outside member countries can licence the system directly. Thanks to its international scope, there are plenty of ways in which Snomed can be customised to local needs. It continues to be developed at every level and takes advantage of the advances that computers and information science have made over the last few decades. In short it is a modern system with the flexibility to adapt and improve.

It is unlikely that you have much choice about which coding system is used for the medical records that you keep as part of your local system. However, much of the success of a system will be down to the people that use it day in and day out. Good data has huge advantages for both patient and clinician, and Snomed can help organise that data, although not on its own.

It does not seem amazing any more that we can ask our phones or other devices to play rock music and get a sensible selection. Underpinning these tools, and Snomed, is simply the computer's understanding of the data that it holds.

Now that we have good reasons to code medical information, let's go ahead and find out more about Snomed CT.

An Introduction to Concepts

Concepts

Concepts are the fundamental building blocks of Snomed CT, although it is actually quite rare that you will meet them directly. As the name suggests, a concept is simply an idea. A concept can refer to just about anything. It is an essential part of all communication to be able to refer to ideas. A concept could refer to our idea of a physical object such as rabbits, clouds or tables, as well as more abstract ideas such as love, dancing or income tax. Very young children would be able to identify the rabbit on the front of this book, even though it might not be identical to other rabbits that they have already seen, because they are familiar with the "concept" of a rabbit.

It really doesn't matter what the concept is or does, as long as we can imagine it. In languages throughout the world we attach names to concepts: we call them nouns. Just as nouns make the foundation of all language, concepts are the basis of all medical coding systems.

Within medical coding we attach labels to all kinds of concepts: parts of the body, micro-organisms, drugs, surgical operations, diseases, laboratory results or anything else that we want to describe. Concepts allow us to communicate our ideas with a good chance that another person will know what we mean.

Most medical coding systems such as Read codes or ICD-10 provide a dictionary of sorts where concepts can be defined. After all, if we can't agree on the meaning then we won't have much idea what the message is about. Definitions can be anything from a few words to a detailed description, but whatever their length, their aim is always to help GPs record and communicate clear and accurate notes without any loss of meaning.

When we code medical information (that is to say, when we record it), we use a standard set of words or terms, a vocabulary, that everyone agrees on. Clinicians, statisticians, management and, crucially, computers can all read and make sense of our notes. So, when we describe a concept, we want to be clear that there is only one possibly meaning.

There are hundreds of thousands of concepts within Snomed CT, and each one describes something different. It is easy to feel intimidated by the volume of information involved: no-one could ever read through all of these concepts, any more than anyone could memorise a dictionary. In practice, however, Snomed's long list of concepts is no scarier than a list of the thousands of buildings, roads or types of flower. We don't need to know all of these concepts: we just want to be able to find concepts we need, when we need them.

Each concept in Snomed CT has its own identifier: a random numerical code up to 18 digits long. The numbers themselves do not matter: they are simply used to distinguish one concept from another.[2]

---

[2] This is a slight simplification. Some numbers can tell you a little about who invented the concept in the first place, but it certainly does not tell you anything about what the concept actually means.

In this sense these identifiers are similar to a person's passport number, or to the barcodes printed on almost everything that we buy. These are an important label, essential when you travel or go through the checkout. The number itself is essentially meaningless. It tells you very little about the product without looking it up in a database.

If you have used other coding systems in the past this can be a little difficult to get used to. Read codes, ICD 10 and others place a lot of meaning on the identifier itself and it can be fairly easy to work out at least some of the meaning from this. Often the code would be printed alongside the text description. You may even have become familiar with some of the identifiers that you used most often. In the other systems, including previous versions of Snomed, codes have tended to be only a few characters in length and it was certainly possible to commit the most common of these to memory.

In ICD-10 the code F03 represents "unspecified dementia" and other, more specific types of dementia have codes that also start with F03. Read codes are similar with codes up to five characters long.

You are unlikely to be able to remember SNOMED CT identifiers, unless you have the sort of brain which can memorise a pack of cards for a party trick. These long numbers are entirely for use by computer programs and you are unlikely to ever see them in a patient record. Instead, what you will see is the text description of the concept that is designed to be read by human beings.

That may be quite a big change to how you work, especially if you have previously used codes for very specific clinical and business tasks such as processing payment claims or classifying cancer diagnoses. In these old systems, similar codes have subtly different meanings, and getting the codes right is essential to prescribing the right treatments and generating practice income. Clinical and financial tasks could become much simpler in the transition to Snomed. If the system is implemented well, it will be possible to rely on the text itself without having to worry that you have picked the "wrong" one.

As medicine has changed through the years, concepts of diseases have changed too. Until about 200 years ago, physicians classified diseases by the four humours of the body: black bile, yellow bile, phlegm and blood. Doctors used leeches were to "balance" the humours by drawing blood from the body. This sounds absurd to us now, but as medical knowledge continues to move forward, things that we now think of as single diseases may soon be found to be several different conditions. Conversely, separate diseases may be found to be different presentations of the same thing. When I trained as a doctor in the 1990s I was taught to distinguish between chronic bronchitis and emphysema. As understanding of these conditions has improved these concepts have now changed – together they are chronic obstructive airways disease.

Previously we could have made a change like this in the coding systems by releasing a new version and asking people to stop using older codes. As I write this the eleventh version of ICD has recently been released. That is a fairly disruptive change, and computers would have to be clear which version of a code was being used in any given message. Updating to a newer edition of a code was a major upheaval and many years could pass between versions, during which time outdated concepts would remain in use and new ones could not be used.

Under Snomed we can mark concepts as inactive if they need to be corrected or are no longer relevant. You can still look them up: we are not destroying any information when we mark concepts inactive; we are simply saying that no new records should be made with these concepts. All of the previous information is still there. There is no need to change or upgrade existing records.

Marking concepts active or inactive is the first of quite a few areas where there is some extra complication to the design of the record system, but making things simpler for users. We no longer have to wade through piles of obsolete concepts when adding information to the patient record. Read codes in the UK have many obsolete codes that are still available for users to enter.

With Snomed, users don't need to worry about accidentally picking inactive concepts as finding the current concept is now Somebody Else's Problem.[3] We will see this again as we explore Snomed CT further – a lot of the work has been pushed onto the authors and maintainers of the concepts working in informatics departments and the developers of the computer systems that we use.

Let's take a breath and see an example using the rabbit on the front cover of this book. Snomed CT

---

[3] My apologies if this turns to be your problem. Good luck - we are all relying on you.

contains a good number of animal concepts so we can code rabbits!

Imagine that we found a rabbit hopping around the consulting room. If we wanted to enter this into our computer system we would use the concept "rabbit" which is associated with the code number 88818001 (but we don't need to worry about the number because it doesn't help us at all). It is an active concept. We would not need to record a dodo so that is not an active concept and we can't use a concept to record a dodo[4].

Snomed is a very flexible system and we can use as many or as few of its features as we want to. We will explore more features throughout this book which together can build very sophisticated record systems. However let's try to imagine a very simple system which uses only concepts.

Using Snomed, we can build a device that only measures one concept: for example, a set of scales that records a patient's weight. When a reading is taken, that concept is recorded along with the measured weight. That information can then be transferred (to clinical system, for example, or printed out for a patient). Snomed does not concern itself with how that information is transferred but now we have a working system using Snomed that will measure weight and enter it into the patient record requiring only concepts. We will build on the foundation of these concepts to see

---

[4] Actually, there is no code for dodo at all: Snomed CT has not been around long enough to need one but if there was a concept it would be inactive.

other powerful tools that Snomed provides but there is a lot that can be done with concepts alone.

Descriptions

Earlier I described concepts as equivalent of nouns in language. The is not the whole story as we still don't have something that we can display in the medical record. There is a code number, which is pretty unhelpful. There is an idea, which is even more difficult to enter or read in a medical record. We need a way to represent the concept in a way suitable for humans to understand.

Let's take the example of the rabbit again for which we have identified a concept. We have already found two ways of representing that concept: the written word "rabbit" and the photograph on the front of this book. I could draw you a picture, make a model, perform a mime or use the sound of the word "rabbit". I could even show you an actual living, breathing rabbit! Having all of these various ways of referring to the same thing is something that is quite normal in everyday life, and we need to have a method of dealing with this variation in Snomed.

Fortunately, for simplicity, Snomed only deals with the written word. There can still be many ways of referring to the same thing. I call it a rabbit but a young child, who can easily recognise it, might call it a bunny or bunny-rabbit. A French speaker would call it *lapin* or a German *Kaninchen*.

None of these things make a jot of difference to the rabbit, who is entirely unaffected by the name that all of these people have been applying to it. It will be entirely unaware of all of this. In fact if we got all of these people together then they could use the rabbit, or at least the idea of one, to help translate from one language to another. The concept of the rabbit remains the same even if the nouns that are used to describe it vary widely. It is the underlying concept that matters and the text that we read is normally an imperfect attempt to describe this.

The same is true in medicine. There is often a common name as well as a medical term for parts of the anatomy or diagnoses. The thigh bone is technically called the femur and the collarbone is the clavicle. Removal of the appendix is also called an appendicectomy, or appendectomy in the USA. It is important that we can reflect this - descriptions are how the language that we use is translated into the underlying concepts that make up Snomed. As Snomed CT is also an international project it needs to be able to cope with all the various languages and dialects that might be used in medical records.

Clinical IT systems do not really care how we refer to a concept, just that the concept remains the same. All of these different terms are simply to help we humans communicate with IT systems and with each other.

Descriptions have their own identifiers in the same way that concepts do. There is even less need for users to know the actual identifiers for these text terms than for the concepts, but you should know that they are there. These identifiers are again of most use to the designers and programmers of medical computer systems. We can also make descriptions inactive if they become outdated, or are found to be inexact or even just plain wrong.

Making a description inactive does not make the concept inactive. It is perfectly possible to have an inactive description of an active concept.

We have already seen that each concept can have many different descriptive terms. Things could rapidly become impossible for users if they had to deal with all of several possible ways and many possible languages for describing a concept. Fortunately, Snomed provides several ways to manage the terms.

Each concept will have a "fully specified name" which gives a brief text description as well as stating what type of concept it is (more about this later on). This tends to be a little formal, like someone using your full name in conversation, and is not normally displayed in the record. At least one other term will be marked as "preferred" and some of the other terms might be described as "acceptable" which are both fairly self-explanatory. For instance, "Flatulence/wind (finding)" is a fully specified name but "Flatulence/wind" is the preferred term internationally. "Farting" is considered acceptable – although you may disagree depending on the context!

One of the ways that Snomed can be customised is to change the list of terms depending on language or context. This allows terms to be specified in the appropriate language or dialect, or just to use the terms that are most suited to a particular clinic or service. There are differences even between the terms used in the United Kingdom and United States editions of Snomed, the most commonly cited being the terms "appendicectomy" and "appendectomy" mentioned earlier but there are numerous other spelling differences.

The term which is presented to you will change depending on which language has been selected, but the underlying concept - removal of the appendix – remains the same. If we are searching for patients who have had appendix surgery, it does not matter which term has been used. We also might have a computerised decision aid for abdominal pain which could rule out appendicitis if the appendix has already been removed without worrying about the exact wording.

Most of the time the term that is entered is the one that will be displayed in the medical record - we generally expect the record to show what we have actually written. Snomed links what is on the screen to the underlying concept.

Using concepts and their related terms we have the basics of a clinical record. This could be entered and displayed on a simple system. Because we have used Snomed it is easily transferred between systems. We don't yet have a way to define any sense of the meaning of these concepts in Snomed but, as we have already seen, Snomed is modular and we can add that function later. In fact that is what we will begin to do in the next chapter.

Relationships

Simple relationships

In the previous chapter we have seen how concepts act as a type of a dictionary. When we use Snomed, the concepts ensure that we are all using the same vocabulary, which is extremely valuable. A measurement of blood pressure or the result of a laboratory test will be clearly and consistently recorded on every system that uses the same concepts. If we want to send a message from one system to the other we know that as long as both systems use Snomed it will be understood. This is the simplest way a computer system could implement Snomed CT. We can also use descriptions to allow us to describe the concepts in any language that we chose. However, if concepts and descriptions were all that was available, we would miss much of the power of Snomed CT.

The system we have described so far is unlike a dictionary in one very crucial way: there are no definitions, other than the text label, that we have applied for human use. A dictionary is more than a list of words and, to a computer the list of terms that we have looks exactly like this.

Some of these concepts will be very similar, such as two types of an antibiotic. Concepts may also be as different as a heart rate measurement and brain surgery. Currently it all looks the same in Snomed.

We have coded our rabbit, but this still relies on us knowing what a rabbit actually is. Computers are notoriously stupid about this sort of thing and can't tell the difference between a rabbit, a hare, a buffalo or even between a heart attack and a measurement of a patient's weight. This is not too much of a problem for cute pets as almost every user is likely to know about rabbits but is a significant issue as we start to describe more arcane medical knowledge.

So how can we describe our rabbit so that even a computer can understand? You might call it an animal. With a little knowledge of biology you could describe it as a mammal. If you were being very general, you might say that it is a living thing. A mammal is a type of animal and both are living things. We could combine all of these together to say that a rabbit is a mammal which is an animal which, in turn, is a living thing.

This sort of description is quite similar to the way that biologists would classify a rabbit within the animal kingdom, down to the exact species. (We have missed out several of the stages for the sake of simplicity). The full formal classification is available within Snomed CT[5] although this is certainly not its primary function. It is always simpler and quicker to use a system that already exists than to invent a completely new one.

You can see our simple classification in figure 2. Each line shows how these are connected. These are called "is a" relationships because, as we work up from the bottom, each concept is a type of the concept above. All

---

[5] Kingdom, phylum, class, order, family, genus and species as every school child has drummed into them.

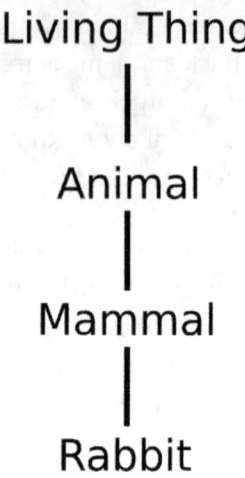

Figure 2: A simple description of our rabbit

rabbits are mammals, for instance. In the jargon of Snomed mammals subsumes rabbits.

We also know that all mammals are animals. Because of the way that these "is a" connections work we can skip over any intermediate steps and say that every rabbit is an animal. We know that if we search for animals we will always get a list of all of the rabbits because a rabbit is a type of animal – missing out the middle step of mammals. In fact the concept of rabbits has an "is a" relationship with everything above it in the diagram. A rabbit is also a living thing. We choose not to put all of these relationships on the diagram to make things neater but they can easily be deduced as we work up the page.

Of course, we want to describe things other than rabbits in our scheme. To be useful we would have to put a lot more concepts in. There is a very simple example in

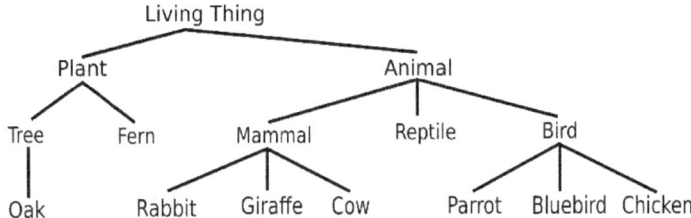

Figure 3: A tree of (some) living things

figure 3. You can see how a pattern develops that looks like an upside-down tree. We don't get any circles because all of these relationships work in one direction only. A rabbit is a mammal, but a mammal is not a type of rabbit. The "is a" relationship will always point upwards. The rule about skipping concepts also remains the same. We can jump as many steps up the tree as we want. An oak is a tree and a parrot is an animal but both are living things.

It looks a little bit like a family tree and each concept can be the "parent" of several "child" concepts. You can see on our tree that each child only has one parent. The terms parent and child are used quite commonly when describing these trees and it can make it easier to remember that these relationships only go in one direction. We can skip generations however. We have been able to say that a rabbit is an animal and that it also is a living thing but the same is true of a cow or giraffe. Parrots take a different route but are still animals and living things but unlike rabbits they are not mammals. Any concept "is a" type of a concept further up the chain. In our family tree it makes more sense to talk about ancestors rather than just parents.

This might seem very obvious but goes a long way to describing what the concepts represent. Because we know that a chicken is an animal then anything we know about animals we know automatically is true about chickens. We only need to tell the system once. Animals move, breath and reproduce and so, by inference do chickens. Mammals have fur and give milk to their young - so we know that is true of giraffes, rabbits and cows without having to spell this out for each individual species.

The top of the tree is currently "living thing" but we could go up further to a "root" concept that covered everything that could be described. This root concept can be helpful when you are designing a coding system but is not very helpful when you are using the system and is generally ignored. The root concept in Snomed CT is "Snomed concept". Every other concept "is a" Snomed concept.

Immediately below the root Snomed concept are some broad chapters for things such as organisms, anatomical features or observations made about the patient. There are also some areas for some of the internal workings of Snomed CT which we will meet later.

We can see this type of division from the general to the specific throughout health care. Hospitals are divided into departments and within these departments staff will have their own interests and areas of expertise. Each will treat a particular set of conditions and perform specific treatments. Sometimes whole hospitals may specialise in a specific set of conditions. Orthopaedic surgeons will deal with bones and ophthalmologists will deal with diseases of the eyes. Amongst the orthopaedic surgeons some may specialise in joint replacements with others treating problems of the spine or hand.

Most coding systems have worked this way to some degree. At the simplest level some have divided their codes into chapters whilst more modern systems have several layers which have allowed quite detailed information about each concept. ICD-10 and Read codes have this structure where each code has one parent and can have a number of child codes.

Sometimes the meaning of the concept will only be made clear by its relationships. Some terms are used in several different ways in medicine. The word fundus, for example, can apply to the stomach, the uterus or several other organs of the body and it may only be by looking at the context to see what the concept "is" that we can understand what it means.

The ability to summarise codes is very important when we come to read the information. We should use a specific code when entering information, but the hierarchy can save us a lot of effort when we are extracting data: if we want to collect statistics about all animals or to trigger an automatic action for mammals we don't have to make an exhaustive list of every creature that possibly fits our criteria. By having a well-defined hierarchy, a lot of the work is already done for us (by those Someone Elses I mentioned earlier). Using specific concepts – near the bottom of the diagram - for data entry and more general concepts – closer to the top - for data extraction we can obtain the greatest benefit from the hierarchical structure of Snomed. In this way we store as much information as possible as well as reading all possible entries when we come to look at the data.

Polyheirarchy

But there is a problem with the hierarchy that I have just described.

The hierarchy works very well if we want to find animals based on their biological classification: for example, searching for mammals will bring up a collection of all the animals which express milk for their young. However, if we want to find all of the animals that are pets, we will need another approach.

The pattern of colouring of the rabbit on the front cover shows that he is a Dutch Rabbit, a domestic breed (which surprisingly seems to have originated in England).

Snomed CT once again comes up trumps with a separate concept for a Dutch Rabbit, which is a type of the rabbit concept. Unfortunately, we are no closer to being able to search for pets. We can't even assume that all pets are mammals as we would miss out goldfish, parrots, tortoises and other more exotic pets.

The problem is, we have the wrong hierarchy. We don't want to define animals based on their anatomy but instead want to see how they fit into the human world. It is not too difficult to create a new hierarchy based on this, certainly if we keep it simple. We can create new concepts for pets or farm animals.

As we have already seen that we move from general to specific as we move down the tree. "Is a" relationships mean that each child concept is a more specific example of the parent concept. In our new hierarchy our Dutch rabbit and perhaps the parrot could be defined as pets. We simply tell Snomed that our rabbit "is a" type of the pet concept.

Chickens and cow are farmyard animals using this way of classifying animals. All of the relationships are still "is a" with each concept belonging to the wider group immediately above it. We could divide things further into common or exotic pets, or add another concept for domesticated animals but this will do for now.

Which hierarchy is better? It depends what we want to do. We have seen that different searches would be facilitated by different hierarchies. This could be a real problem in some coding systems. Unlike a real family tree each concept could only be a child of one other concept. This limitation makes things much easier if you are publishing the codes in a book. It is also fairly simple to represent in a computer system.

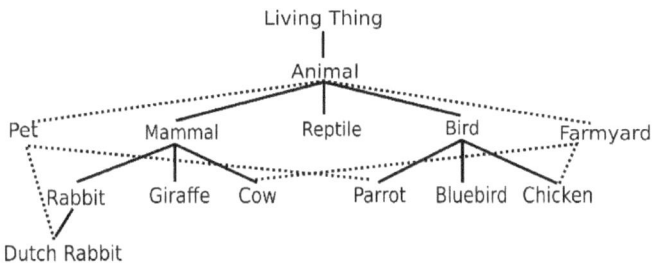

Figure 4: Including a pet based hierarchy

Snomed CT will never be listed in a directory and computers, and their programmers, have come a long way in the last couple of decades and it probably won't surprise you when I say that this limitation no longer applies. Each active concept can have more than one parent although most still only have one or two. Figure 4 shows what happens when we add our new concepts into the tree that we saw in figure 3. The new relationships are shown with dotted lines although they are really no different to all of the other existing relationships.

Branches of the tree they will all join up eventually. Our two hierarchies join up again at "animal". Everything joins together at the root node.

If we draw both of these hierarchies on the same diagram it might seem at first sight that we have introduced a circle which would be a bad thing for "is a" relationships. However remember that each link has a direction so we cannot go around this circle. There are two ways to get from "animal" to "Dutch rabbit" but there is no way back. This is not a circle but more like the way a river runs around a stone — the stream may be split but all the water continues in the same direction.

This is very useful and greatly improves the way that we define concepts: for example, a Caesarean section. Snomed says that a Caesarean section is a delivery of a baby. It is also a significant operation for the mother, and Snomed also knows that it is an operation on the uterus (and by deduction an operation on the abdomen). This will be vital information if the woman needed further surgery in the future.

This sort of hierarchy really starts to make use of Snomed concepts. We can search for quite general concepts, such as any patient who has had a surgical operation or infectious disease, and Snomed allows the clinical IT system to return all the information we need –

even when the records contain much more specific information.

The hierarchy can also be used in data entry. Snomed can use this hierarchy to help suggest suitable terms and concepts based on what is expected. An eye surgeon might see eye operations first and for other data entry, such as laboratory results, the clinician could make only valid suggestions.

Like concepts and descriptions, relationships may change with new editions of Snomed. Relationships can be labelled as inactive as others take their place. This most obviously happens when concepts are added or removed to Snomed but can also happen where there are errors or when general improvements are made.

In the past, asthma was considered a type of chronic obstructive airways disease. Over time this view has changed – that relationship is no longer one that would be considered correct. By making that relationship inactive and adding alternatives this can be updated without ever having to change the patient's record. The patient will still have a record of asthma, but will not be considered to have a type of COPD.

Definitions

These "is a" relationships go some way to defining the meaning of the concepts. By defining a Dutch rabbit as a pet, we have listed one of the ways in which the rabbit is distinct from rabbits in general. It is not completely unique, there are quite a few types of domestic pet rabbit in the world, but we can describe it a little better. The concept of a Dutch rabbit is better defined by saying that it is a pet. There are ways to use this information to help organise data and we will consider this in a later chapter.

What we have not done is added any extra information about the rabbit. We have said nothing about the history of the breed and little about its suitability as a pet. We have not given any information about how to care for the rabbit, for instance what it eats or what time of day it likes to be active. This could be useful information for a pet owner or someone considering looking after a rabbit, so it might be good put some of this in to our coding framework. Coming back to general practice, we might want to say that the antibiotic trimethoprim "is a" treatment for urinary tract infection or that a blood glucose level "is an" investigation for diabetes. This is valuable information for patient care. Presenting this sort of information and advice is often integrated into clinical computer systems where it is called decision support. Surprisingly, Snomed CT doesn't work in this way – and for good reasons. Relationships are not primarily a mechanism to store knowledge, such as at the treatment for a particular condition, but to define the concept better. If the relationship does not add anything to our understanding of the meaning of the concept, and how it differs from other concepts, then it is not included in Snomed. To return to a previous analogy, Snomed is like a dictionary rather than an encyclopaedia, because the management of medical guidance in an international project would be a huge undertaking.

We have already said that a rabbit "is a" mammal, and this particular breed is domesticated because this tells us more about what it is and can help make it clear how it differs from a wild rabbit or anything else. Similarly, we can say that blood glucose level "is a" blood investigation or trimethoprim "is an" antibiotic. These are part of the definition of these ideas.

Decision support and guidelines require separate computer systems, most likely based on local needs and policies. These systems will use the medical record and its data and could use many of the features of Snomed to decide when to trigger support or advice. Medical knowledge databases may well also use Snomed CT codes internally to help them store guidelines, advice or potential drug interactions but their information is not stored directly within the structure of Snomed CT itself.

Congratulations: you have now mastered the basic ideas behind the day to day use of Snomed. Using concepts, their descriptions and relationships, we have the tools to build a very effective system for medical coding with just the ideas that we have seen so far. In fact, a set of codes and the relationships between them has been the entirety of some previous medical coding systems.

Concepts allow the consistent recording of medical information and relationships make the concepts easier to navigate and manage. This is the practical minimum set of Snomed features to implement in a clinical record system and will cover the most data that you might want to deal with.

Snomed has other powerful tools that set it apart from many of the coding systems that have been used in the past and we will explore these later in this book.

Organising Information

Let's take a break from the building blocks of Snomed to start to see how medical information is organised using concepts, descriptions, definitions and relationships.

There has been nothing specifically medical in what we have discovered so far about the structure of Snomed. These tools could be used to describe different types of rocks or pasta recipes as easily as they could information about the medical history of a patient. This flexibility is a great testament to the skills of those people who designed the system in the first place, but we need to put some flesh onto the bones before we have something that will be useful in a clinical record.

There was a little clue about how this information was organised when we talked about descriptions a couple of chapters ago. The Fully Specified Name of a concept will always include the type its concept takes in brackets at the end of the term.

These types are the fundamental concepts on which all other Snomed concepts are built and each is at the head of its own tree. They have exactly one parent (the "root" concept) and each tree is entirely separate – any other concept will belong to one and only one of these trees. (A concept cannot be both a clinical finding and a body structure, for instance).

Some of these types can be relatively obvious and others seem a little more unclear. These more difficult types of concept are generally things that we are quite familiar with but often don't recognise as a different type of thing. These seem unfamiliar largely because we don't name them very often.

Medical records have always had a structure in paper records, long before the advent of computers. A typical entry would record a presenting complaint or diagnosis, medical symptoms and findings from an examination of the patient. The medical history itself would include current symptoms as well as past medical problems. Family history could also be recorded as well as a patient's social history. This could be followed by procedures such as taking blood samples. Later on in the record there could be the results of laboratory tests, X-rays or ultrasound examinations.

Patients may have a surgical operation or other procedure. Much of the time they will be prescribed some medicine and we might also want to record its administration. These different aspects of the medical record are represented by particular sections or subsections of the Snomed hierarchy.

There is a list of the different sections in figure 5. Some of these will be used only in specific circumstances. Others will only be used together with other concepts and are unlikely to appear in the record in their own right. A final group defines the internal structure of Snomed and are only likely to be used if you are developing a clinical record system. This latter group are definitely Somebody Else's Problem.

In the table these concepts are listed in alphabetical order but there is no such thing as a "right" order in Snomed and they could appear in any order on your system. In the next few pages we will meet the areas most likely to be used first and then some of the other areas which support their use.

- Body structure

- Clinical finding

- Environment or geographical location

- Event

- Observable entity

- Organism

- Pharmaceutical or biological product

- Physical force

- Physical object

- Procedure

- Qualifier value

- Record artefact

- Situation with explicit context

- Snomed CT model concept (metadata)

- Special concept

- Staging and scales

- Substance

Figure 5: Snomed CT root concepts

Clinical finding

Concepts in clinical finding to make up a large proportion of codes that you use from day to day, particularly if you are responsible for coding medical consultations. The three crucial pillars of observations, examination and investigation all use codes in this area. These concepts cover everything that can be directly discovered about a patient's clinical state, from the observation of a bruise to a heart murmur or the result of a blood test, X-ray or scan result.

Clinical finding also includes diagnoses, or, "disorders". When you look at a concept such as "diabetes" it will include the word "disorder" in brackets at the end of it. Disorder is classed as a clinical finding. It reflects the idea that most diagnoses are findings about a patient. The authors of Snomed have not been able to come up with any meaningful or useful definition of a diagnosis that does not also define clinical finding. For example, a broken arm is both a clinical finding and a diagnosis, as is emphysema.

This overlap is unlikely to come up particularly often in practice but knowing about it may make searching or analysing data a bit easier.

Procedure

'Procedure' concepts are likely to feature prominently in medical records, second only to clinical findings in the number of times that they are used. Almost every medical procedure is listed, from surgical operations to simply giving some food to the patient. Often the procedure, such as the taking of a blood test, will lead to the discovery of clinical findings. If clinical findings are like nouns in the medical record procedures represent the verbs, describing actions.

Even quite basic things such as taking a clinical history or listening to a patient's heart have their own procedural concepts.

If payments to medical providers are based on the type of care delivered it is likely that these are the concepts that will trigger those payments so there may be a greater pressure to use these correctly than some others. Because of the importance of procedures there has been a lot of attention paid to the creation of suitable concepts, and so this is one of the areas with the most developed model of medical care.

There is a rich hierarchy which provides a clear definition for most of the procedures. We will look at these definitions in more detail in the next chapter.

Situation with Explicit Context

Don't be put off by the name: the concepts contained within this area are likely to prove very useful. 'Context' simply affects how we understand a concept. These concepts have "situation" at the end of the fully-specified name.

If we read "Heart Attack" in a patient's notes we would normally assume that the patient had a heart attack on the date that the entry was made in the notes. This assumes three things: first, that the heart attack happened; second, that it happened to the patient; and third, the time that it happened. If this seems obvious then that is because it is meant to. This is the implicit context and it applies to pretty much anything in Snomed but most specifically to the procedures and findings that we have already talked about.

But perhaps we want to say that the patient has had a heart attack in the past. We might want to say that a patient has never had a particular procedure. We might want to say that an operation is planned for the future or has been cancelled. We could be recording a family history and want to say that a heart attack did not happen to the patient but instead to a family member. All of these are explicit contexts where our usual assumptions about presence, person and time do not apply.

These need their own hierarchy: we can't say that a family history of asthma "is an" asthma - a search would become confused by the change of context. A planned gall bladder operation is not the operation itself.

The context adds to an original concept. One of the largest sections of this area is about family history. A condition here is stated but in the context of another family member such as diabetes in a parent or the death of an aunt.

We can say the same about procedures. A blood test may not have had the results returned yet and this situation can be coded as well. Any concept starting "history of" (or H/O) will appear here as a disorder with a context of the past. That is, we know the condition existed in the past. It may or may not still be present. A history of a broken arm, for example, would likely be healed now.

If you are looking through the Situation with Explicit Context area in a Snomed browser, you might not find as many concepts in this area as you might expect. There are concepts for family history of ischaemic heart disease, but nothing to say if that was a father, mother or great aunt. There is a concept for planned operation on the nose but again nothing any more specific. Don't worry, we can still describe quite specific plans in Snomed and we will see how to do this in the next chapter.

Like almost everything else in Snomed, using the implicit and explicit contexts are optional. Context can be provided directly by the computer system. There might be a location for family histories which can simply contain the finding concepts. In this case we know it is a family history because of how the clinical system records it. Planned procedures may have their own section. There are no rules about how they should be used, as long as the meaning is clear. Snomed provides a way to record this but whether this particular method is used is up to the computer system developer.

Social Context

As the description suggests, Social Context provides a range of concepts that allow us to record information about the patient which is not particularly medical but sits in the "social" section of the medical record. Lifestyle or occupation can be coded using these concepts. In essence these are non-clinical findings about the patient.

There is a subsection for "person" which we can use to record someone's status as a patient, father, Christian, graduate or other factor.

Information may be recorded as part of a clinical history or may be requested to monitor the diversity of groups who access health care. For these reasons this will be a frequently used section.

The remaining sections are not commonly used but they are important when defining other concepts. We will see how they are used in the next chapter.

Body structure

An obvious thing that we might want to code in a medical system is the human body. Much of the rest of our medical records and treatment does not make much sense without a good knowledge of human anatomy.

Human bodies are hugely variable, so our structure will have to deal with all of the possible variations between people. For example, our anatomy changes over time. As we grow bones may fuse together and others extend until they lose the structures that allow them to grow. The concepts in this area are not a description of one human but of all of the things that any human can be.

This is one of the areas where the multiple parents of a concept and alternative hierarchies are very useful: for example, we can describe organs by type as well as by their location in the body using the polyheirarchies that we saw in the previous chapter. The thyroid gland is listed alongside all of the other glands in the body as well as an organ of the neck. The ulna is both a bone and a part of the arm and we can then go deeper to describe specific parts of the bone itself. Its growth plate[6] is both a growth plate and part of the arm. This is an extremely flexible way to describe the body.

Concepts labelled "structure" do not deal with abnormal anatomy. Instead it presents a stage for disease or other abnormalities to take place. Body structure concepts, whilst quite familiar, are not likely to be used

---

[6] The part of the bone that allows it to grow in children and teenagers

directly in a medical record particularly often (for example it does not make a lot of sense to record "finger" in a patient's notes) but these concepts are important due to their relationship to other findings or procedures, which we will explore more fully in the next chapter.

There is a small quirk in the way that anatomy is recorded in Snomed. It might seem that anatomy is a perfect fit for the structure of Snomed that starts from the very general and then moves down to the more specific. It is simple to zoom in from body to leg to knee to the knee cap.

The problem is that this does not quite work. Relationships are supposed to be "is a" and a knee is not a leg any more than a leg is a body. This might seem a bit obtuse, but we can't say that everything we know about a leg applies to a knee or a foot. For instance, we can say that the leg contains thirty bones, but this certainly isn't true of the knee.

The solution to this is to talk about parts of an organ. Part of the foot "is a" part of the leg. A part of the toe "is a" part of the foot (and in turn a part of the leg). Sometimes these "part of" descriptions use terms such as "ankle structure". As we go down the line each anatomical structure is a part of the one above, and in turn part of all the others further up the chain.

What if we want to talk about the foot as a whole? After all, it still exists, even if we can't fit it into our pattern. All we need to do is to say that the whole foot is part of the foot, just a very big part! Nothing else "is a" foot. Toes, for example are a foot structure – alongside, not below, the entire foot. This takes a little getting used to but the general rule of putting as much detail into data entry and searching as high up the structure as possible continues to work well.

Morphological abnormality

This is a separate sub section under body structure. This contains all of the things that, in general, are not meant to be there. In medical terms this means pathology rather than the anatomy of the body. Everything from scars to cysts and tumours will be in here although the location on the body is not defined.

At this stage, there's not much to note about morphological abnormalities, except that entries in this category (for example, pimples) require other concepts to describe size and where that concept can be found on the body.

Observable entity

There are many things that we can observe or measure about a person. In Snomed, observable entities are not the observations themselves but things that can be observed.

For example, we can measure blood pressure, but this is a clinical finding which we have already talked about. In fact, the measurement of blood pressure is actually a procedure to produce an observation. However, when we ask "What is being observed?", the answer is blood pressure – an observable entity. Another example: eye colour is an observable entity, but if we wanted to say that a patient had blue eyes then that is a clinical finding.

Not every observable entity will have an observation concept so they may sometimes be used directly. For example sweat volume is an observable entity but the there is no corresponding finding. It tends to be the less commonly used concepts that don't have a finding concept but if you have the choice it is likely to be the clinical finding that you want.

Environment or geographical location

This is how a physical place can be specified. This can either be a general description such as "hospital waiting room" or can be a specific place. Snomed CT does not contain a particularly large gazetteer and there is not a lot of detail. The USA, for example only has concepts down to state level. In England counties are given while in Australia only the territories are listed. Whilst geography seems like there might be a nice hierarchy it has similar sorts of problems to those we saw in body structure. We can't say that California "is a" United States of America. The structure is however less neat here and states or regions are in a separate hierarchy to countries. The result of searching for the United States will not include concepts entered for California or Texas although this could change in the future.

This is not just about world geography, it also lists types of places. Intensive care units or outpatient departments can be specified, or even the hospital toilet. Outside the hospital Snomed can specify parks and farms, as well as the hopefully more commonly used general practice surgery.

These concepts can be used to describe if an accident happened on the road, or in the kitchen. These could require very different responses.

Geographical concepts would be useful when assessing the risk of infection in a patient according to where they had travelled in the past or which vaccinations they might need based on their future travel plans.

Event

It might seem a little obvious to say that an event is something that has happened to a patient. This is not about medical procedures (they have their own branch) but instead describe the history of the patient. There are not that many concepts in this area and they are a fairly eclectic range including fire, flood, earthquake, and new sexual contact. There is a selection of events about poisoning. The concepts here are only about general types of event – there is no concept for specific events such as the Second World War or Christmas.

A particularly useful concept that will apply to us all eventually is death. There are various child codes about whether the death was: for instance, natural or at the time of surgery. In general, the cause of death is not listed, although for some reason there are specific concepts about fire, electrocution, drowning or overwork.

If you can find a specific event that seems useful they are reasonable to enter in a record. The most commonly used is likely to be death (there is no birth event); searching for other events is likely to be fruitless.

Organism

Organisms are simply living things. The concepts include everything from a whale down to a virus although the latter is more likely to be useful in a medical record. There are many viral concepts and only a single whale concept. This is also where we would see the concepts for types of rabbit that we met in previous chapters.

These are references in the same way as the geographical locations that we saw earlier and are not a way to extend Snomed into veterinary medicine. These are here to help classify the causes of diseases. There is a separate veterinary extension to Snomed which aims to allow the concepts to be used in the care of animals. It will follow the same principles that we have already seen but the details are beyond this book.

Pharmaceutical or biological product

This area is about actual presentations of medicines or other products. This can cause some confusion as some of the terms are identical to the substance area below. When Snomed talks about product it is the physical thing that you can pick up from the shelf. There is, of course, quite a close relationship between the two but, to avoid confusion, it is important to be able to talk about them separately.

A bag of sugar is a product with one ingredient - that is sugar, or sucrose in the more technical terms of Snomed. Both the product and the substance can be called sucrose. However, the bag of sugar could be granulated, caster or icing sugar - each has particular physical properties despite being the same substance. It will also have a particular weight and packaging. This is what makes it a product rather than a substance.

In practical terms most of the codes that are used from day to day are likely to be products. Patients are prescribed products such as antibiotic tablets or an influenza vaccination. These are the concepts most likely to appear in a medication list. Substances, such as penicillin or morphine are unlikely to be coded directly but may be used to describe allergies or adverse reactions. The terms may seem identical for both and differences only become clear when you can see the fully specified name with the area in brackets at the end. This is one area where a good concept browser or user interface will guide the correct use of concepts and prevent significant problems later on.

Substance

Most commonly substances mean drugs, although these concepts stand for chemicals rather than products. Penicillin appears in this section, but tablets, capsules, powders or other specific forms of the antibiotic are listed in the Pharmaceutical Product section.

These may be used in the recording of allergies or to help other systems to monitor for potential drug interactions. In these cases, it is the substance that is important and not the product in which it is delivered.

Physical force

Physicists would say that there are only four fundamental physical forces. Snomed has many more concepts and but only lists two of those that the physicists would recognise. This area contains everything from friction to an explosion. These are very unlikely to be used directly but are likely to be used to describe other concepts, such as trauma or procedures more fully.

Qualifier value

We will talk about qualifiers and their use in more detail in the next chapter. These are the adjectives in

Snomed and has concepts such as left and right, hot and cold, as well as many other ways that we can add to the meaning of other concepts. There are a large variety of concepts here, the most commonly used are probably left and right. Mostly Snomed does not have a completely separate set of concepts for the left and right body structures or procedures - instead we use modifiers to add this information to existing concepts[7].

Record Artefact

Concepts here are parts of the medical record: a record of a physical examination or a written report composed for a patient's employer. This is the scaffolding of a medical record, although Snomed itself does not suggest any particular structure for the record. Clinical systems could use these concepts to allow structured medical information to be recorded: for example, there are concepts for a comment on a pathology result, or an inpatient nursing record. With properly coded records it should be easy to use filters see all of the clinic records or radiology reports for a patient.

These are headings and concepts that have been used in medical records for a long time before computers appeared on the wards and that many of us have used without really thinking about them. As they are used to describe the record itself rather than information about patients, they are likely to be mostly used by informaticians rather than by clinicians.

---

[7] Actually, the US edition does use some separate concepts for left and right, which is entirely compatible with other editions

SNOMED CT Model Component

As well as describing patient care Snomed also describes itself. The concepts in here are used to describe other concepts and we will discuss these more fully in the next chapter. These will not be used on their own.

We have come across some examples already. There are concepts for the terms which we use to describe concepts in plain, human readable language. There are child concepts for the fully specified name as well as synonymous terms. The "is a" relationship has its own concept. We will meet some more soon.

Special Concept

There is not a "miscellaneous" section to Snomed. Instead we have Special Concept which is largely the same thing. Most of these are actually labelled as "Navigational Concept".

Specimen

This section is pretty much what it says. If it is taken from a patient and put into a pot it will appear here. These concepts are therefore most likely to be used in pathology departments to describe the material that they receive from other clinicians.

Staging and Scales

There are lots of grading scales used in medicine. These can vary from stages of cancer to scales used to try to quantify feelings of depression. These are a form of examination for the most part, either directly of the patient or by some other investigation. The actual value or stage will appear as an Observable Entity. The concepts in this area are the scales themselves, not values of quantity such as the level of sodium in a blood sample.

A parallel might be wind strength. Wind speed is simply a measurement and, in the language of Snomed would be considered as a finding. There are specific grading scales of wind such as the Beaufort scale. Other classifications include "gale", "hurricane" or "typhoon" which are recorded alongside the numerical speed. These scales would appear in this area measuring the observable entity of wind speed to produce a finding.

Defining and Creating Concepts

Defining concepts

The types of concepts listed in the previous chapter would seem to be pretty comprehensive. In fact, they might seem to be a little too comprehensive. If you want to see how useful a given concept will be in a patient record, try imaging that concept on a piece of paper with the patient's name and a date or time.

A piece of paper that just said "David Jones - Heart surgery 5th April" would be useful as would one listing the patient's blood pressure, a laboratory investigation or even a diagnostic term such as "type two diabetes". It is more difficult to see how the concepts of "elbow" or "E. coli" could be useful. If the piece of paper was a medication record (and we could identify it as such with a Snomed record artefact concept) then it might be helpful to read "penicillin capsule", but even then it is difficult to see the point of having a concept for the chemical penicillin itself.

Alternatively, despite the hundreds of thousands of concepts which are part of Snomed CT you may want to code something that you can't find a concept for. In fact, there are not even separate concepts for breaking your right or left leg. We seem to have both too few and too many concepts in Snomed at the same time. What is going on?

Let's look back at our rabbit and see how all of these concepts can help us when creating and using a medical record.

It is important to care for your pet rabbit (or any other pet) so we want to make sure that it is being fed properly. We can use Snomed to record that we have given some food to the rabbit.

Snomed classifies this a procedure. Procedures don't have to be medical. Anything that is done will be a procedure and there is a concept for "provision of food", which is exactly what we want. Although Snomed is not a veterinary coding system we can imagine various child codes such as "provision of food to a dog", "provision of food to a cat" and – the one that we would be looking for – "provision of food to a rabbit". Snomed knows that each of these "is a" provision of food. However, the computer cannot say why these are different from each other. As humans we can read the term, but that text is largely ignored by the computer.

This is not a disaster. These concepts are still very usable in a record of pet feeding. Snomed has lots of concepts which are designed in exactly this way. They are described as "primitive" and quite often they can't be avoided. However, we can do a bit better.

One way that we can tell the difference is to use other "is a" relationships. We could have a concept of "procedures on cats", "procedures on dogs" and so on. As each concept can have more than one parent our concept for "provision of food to a rabbit" could be both "provision of food" and "procedure on rabbit". Our new concept would have the features of both and could be considered to be well defined. In fact, we have said about as much about this concept as we need to and can call it "fully defined". In Snomed jargon, that does not mean that we have defined absolutely everything about the concept: just that we have said enough so that it is different to all the other concepts, except its children. In fact, we can say that anything that is both a provision of food and a procedure on a rabbit is, by definition, a child concept of "provision of food to a rabbit".

This is exactly how Snomed defines some concepts. There is, for instance, a concept for cholecystectomy, the removal of the gall bladder. Often this operation is performed without having to make a long incision by using instruments and a camera inserted through the skin called a laparoscope. There is a concept for a laparoscopic procedure which we can use to define the concept for a laparoscopic cholecystectomy. Its definition is simply that it is both a cholecystectomy and a laparoscopic procedure.

If we want to find out about the operations performed in our hospital we could easily search for all gall bladder removals, however the operation was performed. We can just as easily find out about all of the laparoscopic procedures undertaken, wherever on the body they occurred. This is a very powerful feature for writing searches.

We can, however, take things a bit further. At the moment we have some terms that we understand but Snomed still does not. In the surgery, Snomed does not really know what makes a laparoscopic procedure different from any other procedure. We have simply said that some procedures are laparoscopic and others are not but not how they are different.

Going back to our pet feeding example a related problem is that have had to create procedures about every animal. If we wanted to make observations about animals as well this would need a whole further structure and, as they are in separate sections, we can't connect one with the other. We have no way of looking at rabbit procedures and observations together. We seem to have got as far as "is a" relationships will take us.

For humans these might not seem to present many issues. If we are wanting to ask computers to make suggestions or decisions based on the data, we have to be more explicit in defining concepts.

To solve these problems Snomed uses other kinds of relationships. The "is a" relationship that we have used so far is simply a special type of relationship and there are many other relationships that we can use. These are not like the parent-child type relationships that we have already met. They do not generally have the same tree structure - these relationships only go a single step and are about creating a definition of a concept. There are many of these descriptive relationships although only a few are used for each concept.

If I was describing a rabbit I might use its colour, ear type or hair length. None of these things make a lot of sense in a hierarchy but simply act to describe that rabbit more fully.

In medicine, a clinical procedure has a site, a method and an access device. A disease could have a cause as well as a pathological process, such as inflammation. These relationships are not there as a diagnostic aid, but they can allow us to find concepts that we don't know the exact term for. Essentially describing a syndrome could find it automatically.

For the laparoscopic cholecystectomy procedure that we mentioned earlier, the site is the gall bladder, the method is excision and the access device is a laparoscope. Whenever a procedure fits these three criteria it is, by definition, a laparoscopic cholecystectomy. We don't need to find the right concept ourselves as we are entering the data. The computer can infer that based simply on our definition.

We can also use these definitions when applying rules or searches to patient records. We always make sure that we have a report from a pathologist whenever something is removed from a patient. Using Snomed, it is relatively easy to see which patients have had something removed by searching for whoever had a procedure that was an excision. The excision could be anything from the removal of a mole to surgery on a brain tumour. These procedures are unlikely to be close to each other in a conventional coding system but Snomed makes them easy to find.

Relationships are extensively used in the "situation with explicit context" hierarchy that we have already met. We might want to define "family history of ischaemic heart disease" in order to judge a patient's risk of heart disease. This is difficult to do with "is a" relationships – a family history of heart attack isn't a heart attack itself. Instead we say that we have a situation with a subject relationship (a family member) and associated finding (ischaemic heart disease).

This can also be used to alter the time of a procedure, either in the past (history of) or a future planned procedure. A planned cholecystectomy would have an associated procedure (cholecystectomy) and a procedure context (planned).

We can even change the meaning to the complete opposite. If we have asked the patient and there is no family history, we can make this explicit by using the same codes for subject relationship and associated finding but adding that the context is "known absent". The normal, implied, context for Snomed is that the concept is present, so we don't need to say that every time, but we can change it if we need to.

We can even group these relationships together. A common procedure is to remove a cataract and insert a new, artificial, lens in its place to allow the patient to see clearly. This is an operation of two parts. We can use relationships to say that this procedure has a method of surgical extraction but also that it has a method of surgical insertion.

But if we just use the relationships on their own it will not be clear which is being inserted and which is extracted. The solution is simply to group the relationships together so that the extraction is clearly of the cataract and the insertion is of the new lens. This system of grouping relationships together can be used anywhere in Snomed but is principally to be found where a single procedure has more than one part.

This whole system of additional relationships could seem unnecessarily complicated. Why add these other types of relationship to define family history or an operation that has not even happened yet? It makes everything very neat, but what practical benefits are there?

The answer comes down to being able to reuse all of the relationships that we already have. Remember that using "is a" relationships we can always substitute a concept from further up the chain. So we know that a family history of ischaemic heart disease is also a family history of heart disease more generally. We also know that a history of disease in a person's father is also a history of disease in their parent or, more generally, an immediate family member. All of this is automatic where there are defining relationships. These are called inferred relationships because the computer has been able to deduce them based on the stated relationships created by human authors.

If we know that a patient is due to have a laparoscopic cholecystectomy on a particular day, then we also know that they will be on the list of patients who are due to have a laparoscopic procedure. Stores could be automatically checked to make sure that the correct equipment was available.

In some other coding systems there could be several similar codes or concepts and care needs to be taken to avoid selecting the "wrong" one. This is a lot easier in Snomed as the computer can work out if a concept "is an" example of another. For instance, we can say that a patient has a fracture in the leg then they have a broken leg. If we describe a fractured tibia (shin bone) then that looks different at first glance. However, because Snomed knows that a part of the tibia "is a" part of the leg then the computer can automatically deduce that a fractured tibia is a broken leg. As long as we are accurate when putting data into the computer then much of the hard work can be done without needing any manual input.

Where a concept can be described purely, and uniquely, in terms of relationships to other concepts it is called "fully defined". These are seen most often in the procedures and clinical findings areas of Snomed. We can use fully defined concepts to define other fully defined concepts but they must have unique features of their own. Fully defined concepts need more effort to create but like so many of the more complicated aspects of Snomed, that is Someone Else's Problem. As users we get all the advantages of easy to find concepts that the computer can use to make intelligent deductions.

Most concepts in Snomed are not fully defined, although the number is increasing. Concepts which are not fully defined are described as "primitive". They might have only "is a" relationships or might have some other defining relationship. But a primitive concept cannot be defined by a unique set of relationships and it relies on the human operator knowing what is meant. That is not a failure: we cannot continue to define concepts endlessly in terms of other concepts. We cannot give a rigorous definition of a leg, for example, purely in terms of other concepts.

Each concept which has an "is a" relationship with another concept will inherit all of the defining relationships of that concept. In our earlier example we could deduce that, because a laparoscopic cholecystectomy "is a" cholecystectomy and that a cholecystectomy is an operation to remove the gall bladder then we can infer that a laparoscopic cholecystectomy is also an operation to remove the gall bladder. This is called an inferred relationship and can be exceedingly useful.

One advanced feature that flows from this is that every fully defined concept is defined by a unique set of relationships to primitive concepts. This set of primitive relationships is like a fingerprint for the concept. As you move up the tree you will eventually hit a primitive concept.

There can often seem to be more than one way to define a concept using different combinations of relationships. However you do this, if the meaning is unchanged then that fingerprint will stay the same. By comparing these fingerprints, a system using Snomed can make sure that no two concepts have the same meaning.

Making new concepts

Snomed relies so heavily on relationships to define concepts that we need many other concepts describing anatomy or processes of disease. These are not to be used directly but are only used to define other concepts. For example, an entry of "heart" or "inflammation" in a medical record only makes sense if it is related to other concepts. Essentially, we have answered the question of why there seem to be too many concepts. The other question asked at the start of this chapter was why there seemed to be fairly obvious things that did not have concepts. There are concepts, for example, for various types of broken arm, but there is no separate concept for whether it is the left or right arm that has been broken. This would be pretty useful information to have and it is essential if an operation or other procedure is planned.

Similarly, we can say that a patient has a family history of diabetes but there are no concepts to say whether it is a parent, grandparent, brother or sister that has the disease. Many diseases have a genetic component and so we know exactly which family member we are talking about to produce a genetic tree.

Even when making a diagnosis or giving the result of a lab report, the details of a patient's disease can be much more varied than we have concepts to describe.

You may well already have guessed that the answer to these problems lies in the descriptive relationships that we have already met. It is not a great leap to see that we could use an existing concept and add a new relationship. For instance, in the case of a broken arm we could use the relationship "laterality" to say whether it is the left or right arm that has been injured.

We don't have to stop there. The qualifiers section of Snomed contains a wealth of concepts that we can use to refine what we mean. We can say when a measurement was made, for instance, before or after dialysis. We can use other sections of Snomed to pin down a family history to one specific relative. A history of heart disease is rather more relevant when it is your father rather than your great aunt that is affected. Using concepts together in this way means that we don't need to have separately defined concepts for each and every possible combination of illness and family member.

There are even qualifiers for the numbers up to twelve, although these are likely to be less useful than simply using actual numbers as qualifiers.

Let's look at what this means for rabbits before looking at some of the specific medical uses. We have already seen in previous chapters that Snomed has a concept for a rabbit and a child concept for Dutch rabbit. These are both primitive concepts in Snomed as there is not a lot of need for a full description of either in a medical terminology, but it would not be too difficult to define a rabbit if we needed to. A Dutch rabbit "is a" rabbit and this might be defined further by describing its black face, white shoulders and black hind section.

Perhaps one day you come across another rabbit of a completely new breed that has never been seen before. In other coding systems we might just use the concept of "rabbit" as the nearest equivalent. ICD-10 uses codes like "rabbit NEC" – not elsewhere classified – when we don't have a better definition. Using Snomed however we can use the concept of rabbit with extra relationships. Perhaps this new breed of rabbit has long blue fur. We can imagine relationships for length of hair (long) and colour of fur (blue).

What we have done here is create an entirely new concept for our new breed of rabbit. It does not have its own identifier or description like the concepts which are already built in to Snomed but it is every bit as real. We are not limited to those concepts which the authors of Snomed thought should be included. We can make our own. In fact, every time that we describe a left or right wrist fracture we are also creating a new concept.

You might be thinking that these concepts sound similar to the fully qualified concepts described in the previous section and, if you were, then you would be absolutely right. It is simply that fully qualified concepts have been created in advance; in the jargon of Snomed these are 'precoordinated'. New concepts, which we have created as we have needed them, are called 'postcoordinated'. In both cases there are pre-defined rules about which relationships make sense for which types of concept. For example, a procedure can take place on a site, but this must be a body part and not, say, a geographical location. Like constructing a sentence, there are rules of grammar when we are putting together concepts.

These new concepts that we have created will have all the same rules as concepts included in the released versions of Snomed, although they will not have their own descriptive terms. Their relationships with other concepts will give them a "fingerprint" in the same way as pre-defined concepts. There is no risk of duplicating a concept that already exists as the computer would be able to use the fingerprint to spot this easily. The computer can also work out some "is a" relationships if there are any to be found. This means that postcoordinated concepts should be as easy to search for as precoordinated concepts.

Postcoordination is a pretty advanced feature and is much more complicated to implement in a computer system. Normally I would say that this is Somebody Else's Problem and not worry too much about it but in this case it is such a large problem that you may well find the system that you use does not fully support it.

This is particularly likely to be an issue where an existing system has been updated to use Snomed or has only a limited range of functions. Rather than an all or nothing approach, there may be only a few ways that you can modify a concept – for example, by specifying left or right or perhaps listing which family member suffered from a particular disease.

This would be a pity because there is real practical use for postcoordination. You may not have stumbled across a new disease, but existing diseases may occur in an unusual part of the body or a patient's social circumstances may be more complicated than was anticipated by Snomed's authors. This is likely to be the case particularly in specialities like pathology where specimens have to be described or in surgery where an operation is unique to a patient's personal situation.

There are a limited number of family history concepts already in Snomed and so it is useful to be able to construct these as needed. If we want to record a history of plague in a great aunt there is, unsurprisingly, no ready-made concept. Postcoordination allows us to use the family history concept with an associated finding of plague and a subject relationship of great aunt.

That is not to say that without postcoordination there is no use to Snomed. As we have progressed through the features in the chapters of this book we have seen that there are many ways in which Snomed can be implemented but also that each feature brings its own advantages. Snomed is not an all or nothing approach and can be implemented in many ways, as we will see in the next chapter.

Finding Concepts

The main advantage of a well-structured electronic patient record is that we can navigate and find information much more easily than we could if the records were held on paper.

We can search a patient's record for every blood pressure measurement that has been taken or for each instance of surgery that they have had on their heart. A general practitioner could identify every patient who had been prescribed a particular drug if it had been withdrawn from sale. Hospitals might want to know how many operations are planned.

There are two parts to any search. First we have to define which concepts are relevant to our query and secondly we must look for when these concepts occur in the patient record. It is the first process that Snomed can help us with.

A simple way to find the concepts that we are interested in would be to pick an existing concept. We can then use this to find all of the appropriate concepts. Picking "operation on heart" would allow Snomed to select all each concept that is a heart operation including the repair of a heart valve or the removal of a clot.

For other searches we might have to use other types of relationships. If we wanted to find out which patients had been prescribed penicillin then we could use relationships to find all products that had an "active ingredient" of penicillin. The computer would then use that list of products containing penicillin to interrogate the patient records.

It is possible to use several relationships at once. If we wanted to find endoscopic operations on the abdomen we could specify that the concept must be an abdominal operation but also that it must use an endoscope.

This is very similar to the way that we have already defined concepts in this chapter. Snomed can work out all of the concepts that are subtypes of the definition that we have created. Internally Snomed uses something called Expression Constraint Language to create these definitions. The name arises because it is made up of a series of rules that a concept must satisfy to be included. In its most terse form it is based on a mix of mathematical symbols and punctuation marks similar to computer programming languages.

Expression Constraint Language offers a lot of flexibility over simply defining a concept. We can specify a specific concept or only its children. We can combine concepts so say, for example, that an operation must involve the head or a foot, or even both.

We can say that a medication must contain a single active drug, or be a combination of several. We can even say that specific relationships should be excluded from the final result – if perhaps we wanted a list of stroke concepts that did not cause bleeding in the brain.

You are unlikely to meet Expression Constraint Language directly but the principles of using defining relationships to search for Snomed concepts in patient records will be one that you could be using regularly.

Exploring Snomed

Let's look at how these relationships appear in real concepts. There is a list of online Snomed browsers at the end of this book but for this example I am using the one from Snomed International as it has plenty of detail.

To find it just go to http://browser.snomedtools.org and accept the licence agreement. You can then choose an edition of Snomed to use. I am using the International Edition in this example although the details will not be very different whichever edition you choose. We will discuss what a local edition is in the next chapter.

Using the search box we can look for "laparoscopic cholecystectomy". A number of concepts appear with the top suggestion being "Laparoscopic cholecystectomy (procedure)". Clicking on this brings up the details on the right side of the screen. Most of the useful information is contained in the summary tab shown in figure 6.

The box with the dark background displays the core features of the concept that we met in chapter two. At the top is its Fully Defined Name along with the Snomed CT identifier (SCTID) number. That box also contains the other preferred and acceptable terms for that concept. These terms may vary between editions according to the language that is used.

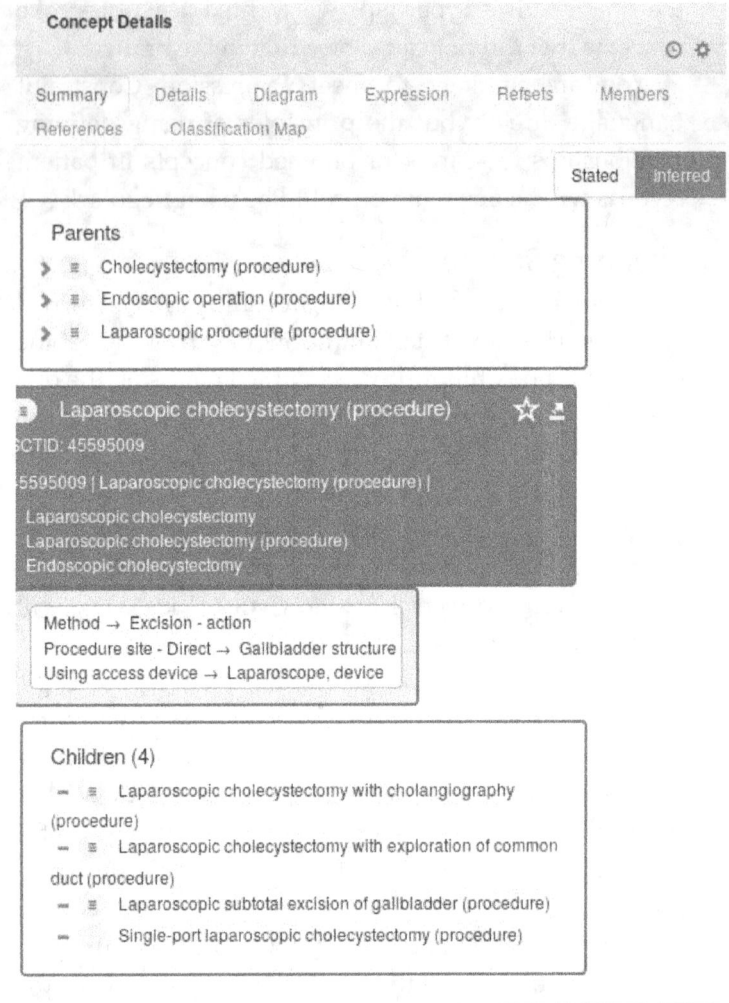

Figure 6: The concept details for laparoscopic cholecystectomy in the Snomed International browser

The other boxes contain the relationships of Laparoscopic Cholecystectomy that we have met already. The top box shows that it has three parent concepts – this operation is a cholecystectomy and an endoscopic operation as well as being a laparoscopic procedure.

It has several children which refer to particular types of laparoscopic cholecystectomy or operations where it has been combined with another procedure. Each of these concepts is a laparoscopic cholecystectomy.

Each of the parent and child concepts is listed by its Fully Defined Name and you can see they are all in the Procedure section of Snomed as you would expect. Each concept also has a yellow blob to its left. If the blob contains three horizontal lines (the "hamburger" icon) it indicates that the concept is fully defined. If the blob is empty then that concept is primitive.

We can see that the laparoscopic cholecystectomy concept is fully defined. The final box on the page contains these defining relationships. In this case the method, site and access method are defined – this procedure is the removal of the gall bladder through a laparoscope.

There is a lot of information here, and this is more than you would expect to see in a clinical system. However it does give a good understanding of how the concept is defined and how you might search for it.

There is one more feature on the summary tab which is less immediately useful but gives an interesting insight into Snomed CT. In the top right corner is a button to select either "stated" or "inferred". Most of the time it is most useful to look at the inferred relationships.

Stated relationships have been explicitly defined by the authors of Snomed. This is how information is added to Snomed. In this case the only parent concept to have a stated relationship is "endoscopic procedure".

I mentioned earlier in this chapter that we can use the rules of Snomed to make some automatic deductions. These are the inferred relationships and are most useful with fully defined concepts.

We can see how this happens in practice here. Because we have defined a laparoscopic cholecystectomy as the removal of the gall bladder then Snomed can infer that this must be a type of cholecystectomy. That might sound obvious to us because of the name but remember that Snomed does not use the descriptive terms at all when making these inferences – it only uses a concept's relationships.

At the same time, we have also said that it uses a laparoscope, so it must also be a laparoscopic procedure.

The same applies to the child concepts. A single port laparoscopic cholecystectomy is a primitive concept but because it has the defining relationships of being the removal of the gall bladder with a laparoscope then it must also be a laparoscopic cholecystectomy.

These inferences are made before each release of Snomed and, to the user, there is no difference between a defined and an inferred relationship. This is a real and practical benefit of Snomed's logical model.

Only concepts that appear in a release, i.e. precoordinated concepts, can have the inferred relationships included in the release. However, postcoordinated concepts which are generated as data is entered in the patient record can have exactly the same sort of inferences made about their relationships to other concepts based on their defining relationships.

It is worth taking some time to have a look around Snomed and the concepts that you might use from day to day. There are a variety of online browsers available and a selection are listed at the end of this book. Now that you know how concepts are defined you can see how these definitions are put into practice.

Moving to Snomed

Mapping

In the previous chapters we have seen that Snomed CT is capable of storing almost every part of a patient record: observations, procedures and investigations from before birth until death. It can be searched easily and even understood automatically by certain computer systems, making life easier for clinicians and safer for patients. It all sounds wonderfully simple.

In real life, however, things tend to be a bit more complicated. There is already a lot of information in digital records, and much of this will have been coded in a framework other than Snomed. Examples might be OPCS for hospital procedures, ICD-10 for diagnoses and Read codes for data on general practice systems, but there are many others. Information on the patient's record may continue to be entered in one of these formats, and data might need to be transferred to other systems – perhaps to produce statutory statistical reports or generate accurate claims for payment. Snomed is not particularly designed to create reports like the Bills of Mortality that we discussed in chapter one. The multiple hierarchies make it easy to double count. For example, if we have separate categories for death by "infection" and "lung disease" then a patient with pneumonia would be counted in both categories. A similar situation can occur with using codes for procedures and operations for generating invoices. Whilst Snomed is comprehensive there will still be a need to use other systems for particular purposes.

We saw earlier that different languages use different words to describe single concepts. The same can be true of different coding systems. Just as a French/English dictionary will tell me that the English word "rabbit" means the same thing as the French word *lapin*, we can use a dictionary to translate between two different coding systems: "maps", in Snomed jargon. Most of the time translation in Snomed is automatic. Maps are available for most of the commonly used classification and coding systems and what's more, this system is constantly updated.

There are always limits when translating from one language to another. A quote attributed (almost certainly incorrectly) to George W Bush stated that "the French have no word for entrepreneur". Whether he said it or not, it is true that sometimes a concept simply does not exist in one of the languages.

In other cases, the concept does exist but not all of the meaning is intact. Eskimos may not have a hundred words for different types of snow, but the English have nearly as many words for rain. It would be surprising if translations for "drizzle", "mizzle" and "squalls" retained their full meaning when translated into a language from a much drier country. Detail gets lost during the mapping process.

Snomed has more concepts than almost any other coding system so it is likely that more problems will be found when translating out of Snomed into another coding scheme. Other systems have been more focused on a single area and so could have concepts that Snomed does not have. Because of this loss of information mapping is not a two-way process, just as human translation is not. Converting one way and then back again will not always put you back where you started.

If I use Google to translate the sentence "My rabbit is frisky and likes to hop around my back garden" into Spanish, the translation is given as, *Mi conejo es juguetón y le gusta saltar de un lado mi jardín trasero.*

If I then ask Google to translate this back into English then the phrase becomes "My rabbit is playful and likes to jump around my backyard." The general gist of the sentence is still there but some of the words have changed. Translation of human languages is not an entirely reversible process due to differences between languages. Spanish may not have an exact translation for the word "frisky" and Google, being American has used the word "backyard" as a term for a domestic garden. Whilst these differences may seem trivial, they may be more significant between coding systems.

Most maps are only designed to be used in one direction and it is not a great idea to be switching back and forward between systems. There can be a degree of loss of information like taking a photocopy: if you take a photocopy of a photocopy the quality is likely to reduce and the quality will deteriorate further as the process is repeated.

The description of a map will not only specify the two coding systems which it will translate but also the direction in which it should be used.

Some maps may use inactive concepts. A common example is likely to be when translating from ICD or related coding systems. These would use terms ending in NOS or NEC –standing for "Not otherwise specified" or "Not elsewhere classified" either where information is not available or a there is no better code. Snomed does not use these but has inactive concepts for the sake of making a smooth transition. It does not matter if some of the current data is translated to these codes - they remain valid and part of the structured record. However, there should not be any inactive codes newly entered in a Snomed based system.

As an aside it is probably worth saying why Snomed does not use Not Otherwise Specified or Not Elsewhere Classified. NOS and NEC codes have largely been used in the International Classification of Disease and systems derived from it. When there is not enough information to use a more specific code in Snomed, we tend to just use a less specific code further up the hierarchy. If we don't know if lung disease is pneumonia or asthma we can just call it lung disease. Not Elsewhere Classified is used when the clinician can't find a concept that fits the diagnosis, and none of the other concepts fit. This does not work with Snomed because in order to say that no other concepts fit, we have to know what all of the other concepts actually are. It is defined by what it is not. There is no sort of definition which would link it to every other concept. An even bigger problem is that, unlike ICD, Snomed concepts can change from time to time as well as from place to place. The meaning of NEC would be different in every case, which is not what we want from a health record.

Concepts are the only element mapped in and out of Snomed. Relationships are specific to each system. When we map one concept in or out of a system, we are translating the meaning and not the context. If a concept has an "is a" relationship with another concept within Snomed, it does not necessarily follow that it is also sub-concept in another system. In fact, it is unusual for concepts to have more than one parent in other schemes and so this will inevitably change when moving across the map. Searches or inferences based on Snomed classifications are unlikely to produce the same results after mapping.

The inverse will also be true. For example, "occupational asthma" is listed in Snomed as a type of asthma. In UK Read codes asthma and occupational asthma belong in completely different sections. Similarly, Read codes have asthma as a subset of chronic obstructive airways disease, whereas they are quite separate in Snomed. For the most part Snomed better reflects current clinical thinking about diagnostics, as concepts can be changed and updated as medical knowledge moves on.

Subsets

Snomed is much larger than any system that has gone before. There are hundreds of thousands of concepts and millions of descriptions. Whilst almost anything can be described with concepts, it is likely that in most situations only a relatively small number of them will actually be relevant at that time. For example, a surgeon is likely to want to describe the operations that they perform but may not be entering much social context whilst in the operating theatre. At the same operation the anaesthetist will record more observations about the patient and the various drugs and fluids that have been used to treat them. The nurse on the ward will not need to describe the operation at all but will need to be able to record observations and procedures such as dressing changes or the removal of drains.

Each clinical role has its own set of requirements for a coding system, so coding works best if everybody agrees on which concept, or group of concepts, will be used in each situation. The record is much more useful if concepts are used in a consistent way. By the same token, there are also many concepts which should probably not be used directly: for example, concepts for "left" or "four" only make sense as attributes of other concepts and will not be used on their own in a medical record.

Snomed allows the use of subsets, which are sets of concepts to be used in specific contexts. These narrow choices down to only the concepts that are needed and make selecting the right concept a bit easier. Subsets are often simply a list of concepts. A more sophisticated way to create a subset would be to give a description and let the computer work out the rest. For instance, we could simply say that the subset will contain surgical operations on the leg and let the details be calculated automatically using the Snomed logic and relationships.

An analogy might be using a paper map. When going out for a walk you will take a map that just covers the area that you will be walking in and features that are likely to be useful to you. It will have footpaths and details of the terrain through which you will be walking. Walkers in other areas will have different maps, although many of the areas covered by the maps will overlap. You would need two quite different maps if you were making a journey by car or sailing a boat. Maps of public transport may look entirely different to topographical maps, containing very few other features other than public transport information.

In Snomed, subsets contain just the concepts that are needed for a given situation. They should not be about restricting choice for the user but simply a way of making Snomed more relevant to what you are trying to do.

Subsets are one example of a more general tool: the Reference Set, more generally known as a Refset. In general, Refsets are where all of the customisation of Snomed goes on. They are used for all sorts of things but it is in the creation of subsets of concepts or descriptions where you are most likely to meet them.

Anyone can create a subset. Some are produced by the international Snomed organisation, along with the main Snomed code list. Each country will have an organisation to manage Snomed in that country and they are likely to produce subsets of their own. Other subsets can be produced by computer system suppliers or even individual organisations, hospitals or departments. As always, it pays to check out what has already been done by someone else but there is a huge amount of flexibility available for a relatively small amount of effort. Using the hierarchies built in to Snomed it can be quite easy to specify an appropriate range of concepts.

However, once they have been created subsets need to be maintained. As Snomed is updated and developed new concepts may need to be added or others removed. Each subset will need a clear plan for its maintenance. This is relatively easy at international or national levels but may be more difficult in smaller organisations as the people who maintain the subset join or leave.

Language

Earlier in the book we looked at descriptions, or different ways of describing a single concept. We can have multiple ways of saying the same thing either with different phrasing (synonyms) or even different languages. The two languages supported by the international edition of Snomed are English and Spanish, with some further support for differences between US and UK English.

Countries and organisations can create their own terms by translating the concepts into other languages or local dialects. There obviously needs to be some care to make sure the meaning is preserved in the translation, but this can be simpler when using technical terms than it would be with general speech or text. With hundreds of thousands of concepts a complete translation is a large task, but by concentrating on the more commonly used concepts and falling back to English or Spanish for other codes it can become a little more manageable. This is most likely to be done at a national level or even internationally where countries share a common language and can work together.

Adding extra terms can be used together with the maps that we met in the last section. If a Snomed concept has a map to a code in another system with exactly the same meaning the text from the older system can be added as a term in Snomed. For users this will mean that they don't see any difference at all in how a concept is represented on their system.

Of course, users shouldn't see all of these terms in every language and there will need to be a way to specify which of the terms should be used in each situation. We can have a list (similar to a subset) of all the terms in a particular language which are preferred for use in clinical records. Once again this is supported by the International Edition for English, but new terms will need their own information to say which should be used.

That can be customised by language, country or even at the individual organisation level.

Behind the scenes these are using Refsets again, just like the creation of subsets.

None of this affects the concepts or alters their meaning so the data recorded is still easy to move between computer systems and different organisations, but we can change how the medical data is displayed to make things easier for individual users. The same concepts will display different descriptions depending on the language selected. This does not add any new meanings in itself although that becomes possible with a different approach.

Local Concepts

Sometimes it seems that Snomed can describe almost everything that there is. Its sheer size seems to make it likely that you could find a concept to describe pretty much anything that you could want to put into a medical record. However, in practical use it is likely that you will find something that you simply cannot find described specifically in a concept.

There are a huge variety of health systems that could be using Snomed and each will have their own requirements. A specific and essential concept in one system may make no sense in another place. Much of this may be around how health systems are organised. There might also be some specific concepts that we want to transfer from a previous coding system using a map as described earlier in this chapter.

In an international project all of the concepts in the main release should be useful and clear in every country of the world.

One way around this could be to make our own concepts. We have already seen that we can create these pretty much at will by the combination of existing concepts. This can be extremely powerful, but it can also be difficult to use. For information to flow from one system to another it would require all of the systems to support postcoordination, which is fairly big hurdle. Even then the concepts will not have a text description to allow users to easily understand them. That is acceptable for specialist care but likely to make things more difficult if the concept is used frequently.

Postcoordination will only create "fully defined" concepts for us. We cannot create new primitives which does put tight constraints on the sort of concepts that can be generated.

As an example, there was, in the past, a form in the UK National Health Service called the FP69. This form was used when the local Health Authority thought that a patient had moved away and should no longer be registered with a particular doctor. As payment to UK general practitioners is largely based on the number of patients registered with their practice this was an important form for both the doctor and the Health Authority.

As records moved to computers so did the forms, and they needed to be described in the medical records. It needs a concept and it would sit quite nicely in the "record artefact" section of Snomed. In fact, there is already a "medical forms" concept for it to be a child of. However there is no concept in the International Edition that would allow the form to be called an "FP69" or give any detail describing the function of the form. We simply cannot make the sort of full definition using relationships that would be needed to create a postcoordinated concept.

As this exists already in medical records we would expect it to be transferred using a map as we move to a Snomed-based system. Things would be much simpler if there was a specific concept. In any case we would want to avoid a large number of postcoordinated concepts as they tend to be relatively unwieldy in the medical record.

This could be added to the International Edition of Snomed but for the majority of countries this concept would make no sense at all. If every country added their own forms then Snomed would become increasingly cluttered with concepts that irrelevant to most users. In general additions to the core of Snomed are only made when they will be understood in the same way around the world.

The solution is simply to let us add our own concepts to Snomed. This is most commonly done at a national level but can equally be done in a smaller region, a particular health system or an individual institution such as a hospital. These additional concepts can be fully integrated into the existing Snomed hierarchy. As we are adding entire concepts these can be primitive as well as fully defined. They will have their own terms and can have relationships to any other concept we wish. We can even add several concepts which are related to each other as well as being part of the overall Snomed hierarchy.

At the national level member countries combine their own concepts with the International Edition of Snomed to create their own National Editions. When you use one of the online browsers you might be asked which edition you want to use. Normally this is a pretty easy decision to make but it is worth being aware that some concepts will not exist in all editions. This may become relevant when transferring data between systems that use different editions. There are ways that automatic systems can help such as using a less specific concept, but this will come down to specific implementations.

Care needs to be taken that these local or national concepts don't duplicate existing concepts from the main international Snomed tree. The identifiers numbers are allocated in a way that means that they will not clash but it is still possible that concept meaning may be duplicated. Avoiding this situation is not as easy as it seems, as new concepts are added to Snomed twice a year and duplication with these novel concepts should be avoided. There needs to be some mechanism to review local concepts regularly to ensure that they remain relevant. Nevertheless, they are an essential aspect that makes Snomed usable in very different environments.

Occasionally a national concept will be promoted to the International Edition, but a concept will never move in the opposite direction from international to national.

Education

I hope that through this book you have seen the features of Snomed that will allow improvements in how data can be entered and analysed within an electronic health record system.

But not everything about moving to Snomed is going to be about the technical details. Whilst a good record using the Snomed system should not put all of its inner workings on show, there are likely to be some visible changes. After all, if everything goes on exactly as it did before then there was very little point in making the change in the first place.

There are real advantages to be had at every level from moving to Snomed. However, the benefits only appear when users enter good quality data. Once a user enters good data – about blood pressure, for example, or height or blood sugar levels – then the system can present this in a useful way. Where there is data about patient allergies and current medication then an electronic prescribing system can warn the clinician if a proposed drug may cause harm to the patient. Decision support systems can use data about the medical history and current observations to present appropriate guidance to the clinician. The purpose of an electronic health record should be to use data to help the clinician treat the patient effectively and safely, although I accept that this is not always the case.

At the wider level Snomed makes it simpler for clinicians to monitor the quality of care. Clinical audit is a vital part of modern medicine: good data and effective tools can make this easier to do and by extension increase its impact on patient care. Systemic problems are easier to see with a better view of the whole system.

There will inevitably be a delay between a clinician entering data into Snomed and experiencing clinical advantages. Many of the advantages require a body of data to work with. Initially there is a time of data entry without beneficial feedback. The old adage of "garbage in, garbage out" applies here. If good data is not entered, then the advantages will never appear.

Data that uses the structure of Snomed will be easy to find again later. If we can record "fracture of the neck of the humerus" rather than just "fracture" then there is much more data that can be used to make sure that the patient gets the best care. If we go even further and code the cause of the fracture then automatic systems can suggest whether this was just an unlucky event or if the patient could have fragile bones.

Implementation of a Snomed system is likely to be a big event at a clinic, practice or hospital, requiring changes to everything from the forms used for data entry to searches and reports. I would suggest that this needs to be done as early in the project as possible. Evidence of real and rapid benefit to those people entering data will be a vital part of ensuring data quality in the new medical record system.

I have often mentioned in this book that various features of Snomed are optional when implementing a computer system. Every system is likely to have its own special features; there cannot be a single guide to entering data. Some systems may use well-defined forms. Others might allow you to search for a specific concept. Advanced systems may interpret free text or even use speech to enter Snomed concepts. Whatever method is chosen, using a modern electronic record will take some training just as writing in a paper-based record does. This is a skill to be learned and will increasingly become an essential clinical competence.

Each system will work differently and a book like this cannot tell you how to use your specific system. What is constant, though, is that it is a vital feature that other people can see and understand what has been written. Education is as important to an effective medical record as any of the technical features of Snomed.

Into the Future

Snomed CT is already deployed in medical record systems around the world. It is used in medical research as well as direct patient care. It continues to be developed and improved. But where will it be in the future?

Technology moves on rapidly and we have new capabilities all of the time. As Snomed descriptions are translated into more languages there is potential to transfer medical records internationally.

This could allow the automatic translation of the records into other languages. Currently English and Spanish are supported by Snomed International but other languages are supported in national editions. As more countries adopt Snomed and produce their own local translations the potential combinations increase exponentially.

Written descriptions of concepts don't only allow human users to understand the concepts that the clinical IT system has stored. They can also be used the other way around.

Computer systems that can read records written in free (uncoded) text are currently under development, which could allow the use of reports or letters written in the past that remain relevant to the patient's medical history. If the computer system knows many of the different ways that we can describe a concept it can use these to understand what has been written in the record. At the moment the technology to automatically convert text to coded concepts is mainly used to help with research projects, but as processes improve systems may become reliable enough to be used for patient care.

As computers become better at recognising speech we could also enter coded clinical data just by talking. We are already familiar with digital assistants such as Siri and Alexa at home and it is not a big leap to the consulting room.

To understand human language correctly, the system needs to know all of the different ways that a concept might be described. Snomed, with its variety of different terms connected to concepts, can help with this. It might be some time before we can rely completely on this language processing as a basis for clinical decision making, but we should expect to see more support for clinicians, as well as audit and management information, from data collected this way in the near future.

Understanding natural language is likely to use some form of artificial intelligence. AI is a term that describes a wide range of techniques allowing computers to make decisions that would previously have only been made by humans. We have already seen that computers can check potential interactions between drugs or advise on which course of treatment is recommended by guidelines.

In the UK, chatbot apps are being used to give a diagnosis and advice to patients based on their responses to questions.

We often hear about machine learning, where a computer has learnt from thousands of images or huge databases of information about people. Essentially the computer is drawing its own conclusions from raw data.

However, intelligent decision support is likely to take a different course. Instead the AI will learn in a similar way to a student doctor or nurse. It will process guidelines and medical textbooks in order that it can produce the correct answer at the right time. The volume of medical evidence currently available is so large that it is hard for a clinician to keep fully up to date. Rather than trying to find new knowledge the AI will attempt to organise the knowledge that we already have.

One of the best know answer finding systems is Watson, which is produced by IBM. In 2011 it won a special edition of the US quiz show Jeopardy against two expert human players. Of course this was simply a demonstration; IBM had bigger plans for Watson, even if they did win a million dollars.

Watson is now being used in medical applications and it is unlikely to surprise you to learn that one of the sources of knowledge that it uses is Snomed CT.

Watson will not only use the descriptions to match medical records to concepts but also the relationships between concepts to make deductions. If it learns a fact about bones it will know that it is true about the femur because the femur is a bone.

Similarly, if it knows a risk of abdominal surgery then it knows that this will apply to both cholecystectomy and caesarean section operations. It will use Snomed to assist both with learning new information and interpreting clinical data about each patient. Watson can link information about the current patient with medical knowledge and records about similar patients in the past to make suggestions and recommendations.

Classify and coding to assist AI systems is common in areas outside medicine. Netflix, for example, has over 3,500 categories of films and TV shows which it uses to try to predict what you would like to see next. Applying these categories is not automatic; computers can't tell a romantic comedy from an action adventure on their own and, as in Snomed, it is people who make the decisions. However, the application of classifications in making recommendations is done entirely by computer.

We are likely to see more clinical systems using artificial intelligence in the future. The application of AI in medical record systems will improve the interface for both clinicians and patients. A reduction in clicking and typing will be welcomed by users.

Ten or twenty years ago computer users were expected to know where their files were stored on their computer. In the 1980s programs would be started by typing in commands on a black screen which displayed little but a flashing cursor. Much of this is now invisible on our phones and tablets and, as users we don't need to know much about their internal workings.

In some ways our record systems are lagging behind but we will be seeing less of the internal mechanisms of medical records as the record develops. The benefits of coded records such as the intelligent presentation of information about the patient and relevant decision support may become almost automatic.

It will be a number of years before AI has a significant effect on clinical practice. Good quality medical records will become even more important as they are used in new ways to assist in patient care. Data will continue to be entered by clinicians but may also come directly from medical devices such as blood pressure machines or laboratory analysers.

There are already AI systems which will analyse medical images such as retinal photographs or X-rays and they may also add data to the medical record using Snomed concepts.

Finally, data coded with Snomed, will be transferred from other clinicians and organisations who are providing care to the patient. Snomed allows these records to be seamlessly integrated to provide a holistic view of the patient's health and treatment, customised to assist the person reading the record.

Even as the coding and classification of medical data becomes less visible to users Snomed will continue to be highly relevant within these record systems as an important way of linking other sources of information together.

All of these technologies exist today although they are not yet widely used and it will take time until they are commonplace in surgeries, clinics and hospitals. I hope that you can use your knowledge of Snomed to make them more effective in delivering care to patients.

Further Learning

If you are planning to implement Snomed or write new content either at a local, national or international level, there are Snomed educational and training resources which are produced for users in the UK, US, Australia and India by local organisations.

You can also find and updated list of these links and those in the next section at https://startingsnomed.com

UK
https://digital.nhs.uk/services/terminology-and-classifications/snomed-ct

USA
https://www.nlm.nih.gov/healthit/snomedct/index.html

Australia
https://www.healthterminologies.gov.au/learn?content=documentlibrary

India https://www.nrces.in

Snomed International owns and develops Snomed CT on behalf of its member countries. Its website (https://www.snomed.org/) contains information and technical documents for Snomed users as well as offering free e-learning courses at all levels.

There is a continually updated list of national resources kept on the Snomed website.

https://elearning.ihtsdotools.org/course/view.php?id=8

Snomed Browsers

There are several online systems that allow you to explore Snomed without implementing it. They have a variety of ways of presenting information about concepts and their descriptive terms. This way of looking at concepts is ideal for exploring Snomed although you would probably would not want to use these types of interfaces in a live clinical system. All of these browsers will require clicking to accept a licence agreement although these should all be fine for personal use.

The official browser of Snomed International is http://browser.snomedtools.org/. This makes a number of different international versions available and you can pick whichever is most useful to you. It is also open source and if you have the time and the skills you can produce your open version of it. It is probably the most authoritative and makes it easy to see all of the properties of concepts, although this can be a little confusing at first.

There is a specific UK version of this browser https://termbrowser.nhs.uk/? which contains the UK edition of Snomed as well as the UK drug extensions. These drug extensions contain concepts describing packs and brands of medicines which are available in the UK.

My favourite browser for looking at "is a" relationships (see chapter 3) is the Shrimp browser ontoserver.csiro.au/shrimp/. This shows concept relationships graphically. The versions or Snomed used principally Australian national releases, although a limited number of UK, US and international editions are also available.

The official browser in the USA is from the National Library of Medicine. It does not have any distinctive features. It requires a free registration.

https://uts.nlm.nih.gov/snomedctBrowser.html

There are many other browsers, some of which you can download to your computer; these are necessarily more complicated to set up. Snomed International keeps a list of currently live browsers on its website at https://confluence.ihtsdotools.org/display/DOC/SNOMED+CT+Browsers

Snomed International official browser
http://browser.snomedtools.org/

Snomed UK official browser
https://termbrowser.nhs.uk/?

Snomed US official browser
https://uts.nlm.nih.gov/snomedctBrowser.html

Glossary

Acceptable – A synonym that is active, but not preferred.

Active – A concept, description or relationship included in the latest release.

Concept – A fundamental unit in Snomed encapsulating the idea which we are describing.

Description – A text description of a concept. Each concept can have several of these.

Expression Constraint – Snomed CT's language which allows searching for a set of concepts using their relationships to other concepts.

Fully defined – A concept that is uniquely defined by its relationships with other concepts. No other concept has the same relationships

Fully specified name – The formal description for each concept, including the name of the concept type in parentheses at the end.

ID – A long identification number for a concept, description or relationship. Has little use in clinical settings.

Inactive – A concept, term or relationship that is no longer in current use. Inactive concepts are not deleted, and remain valid in-patient records, but should be not be used to create new data entries.

Inferred Relationship – A relationship that has been created automatically using existing relationships.

International Classification of Diseases (ICD) – A disease classification system curated by the World Health Organisation. Now at version 11.

International Edition – The version of Snomed produced by Snomed International. All national editions are based on this edition.

"Is A" relationship – A relationship in which one concept is a more specific version of another. Also known as a parent-child relationship.

Map – Used to translate Snomed concepts to and from another coding system.

National Edition – A version based on Snomed's International Edition that contains additions for a specific country.

Postcoordinated – A concept created along with its defining relationships at within the patient record.

Precoordinated – A concept for which Snomed has defined relationships in an official release of its International Edition.

Preferred Term – A description that is preferred for use.

Primitive – A concept that is not uniquely defined by its relationships. Another concept could have the same relationships.

Read codes – A UK primary care based coding system originally designed in the 1980s. Version 3 were known as Clinical Terms and added the 'CT' to Snomed.

Refset – A set of customisations such as lists of concepts and language preferences that any Snomed user can produce.

Relationship – A description of how one concept relates to another.

Snomed – An abbreviation of Systematized Nomenclature of Medicine although it is very rare that the full name is used

Snomed International – The non-profit organisation which own and manages Snomed CT. It was previously called IHTSDO.

Snomed RT – An older coding system which is no longer supported, although is still used, particularly for pathology. RT stood for Reference Terminology.

Stated Relationship – These are relationships that have been created by the developers of Snomed

Subsumption – The process by which one concept encompasses another. Where concept B "is a" more specific version of concept A, A (the parent concept) subsumes B, the child concept.

Synonym – Any description other than the fully specified name.

Acknowledgements

Snomed International put a huge amount of information out detailing every part of Snomed and whilst that is extremely helpful, I must thank David Markwell and the whole of the Snomed education team for guiding me through my first steps with Snomed.

I must also thank Ellie Broughton, who edited most of the text for her many helpful suggestions to make what was in my head clearer on paper.